Table of Contents

Introduction: A Conversation about Home Fitness Success

 Welcome to "Healthy at Home: The Ultimate Guide to Home Fitness Success"! We're so glad you've picked up this book because it's packed with everything you need to know to get fit and healthy right from the comfort of your own home. Whether you're just starting out on your fitness journey or looking to ramp up your current routine, we've got you covered.

Let's face it, life can be hectic. Finding time and motivation to hit the gym regularly isn't always easy. That's where home fitness comes in – it's convenient, flexible, and puts you in control. This guide will show you how to turn your living space into a personal gym, set achievable fitness goals, optimize your workouts, and stay motivated along the way.

First things first, setting clear and realistic fitness goals is crucial. These goals should match your aspirations and keep you focused. Throughout this guide, we'll help you figure out what you really want to achieve and how to get there. We'll talk about everything you need for an ideal home gym, from choosing the right equipment to planning your workout space and ensuring it's safe.

One key to effective workouts is mastering exercise form and technique. This isn't just about avoiding injuries – it's also about making sure you're getting the most out of each exercise. We'll dive into the details of how to perform key exercises correctly, complete with tips and instructions.

Nutrition is another big piece of the puzzle. What you eat can significantly impact your fitness progress and overall well-being. We'll provide advice on how to optimize your diet to boost your physical performance and health.

Now, let's talk about functional fitness. Traditional workouts often focus on aesthetics, but functional fitness is all about improving movements you use in daily life. By incorporating these exercises into your routine, you'll see benefits not just in your workouts, but in your everyday activities as well.

Staying consistent and motivated is essential for long-term success. We know it's easy to start strong and then lose steam, so we'll share strategies to keep you on track and help you overcome any obstacles. A positive mindset can make a huge difference, and we'll show you how to cultivate one.

Recovery and self-care are just as important as the workouts themselves. To avoid burnout and keep your body in top shape, we'll give you tips on incorporating restorative practices into your routine.

Tracking your progress and celebrating your milestones is a fantastic way to stay motivated.

We'll explore different ways to measure your progress and highlight the importance of recognizing your achievements along the way.

Finally, a healthy lifestyle extends beyond just exercise. We'll talk about habits that support overall well-being, like managing stress, getting quality sleep, and developing a positive relationship with food. A well-rounded approach will enhance your physical, mental, and emotional health.

This book is your all-in-one guide to achieving optimal health and fitness from home. By following the principles and strategies we've outlined, you'll build a strong foundation for long-term success. Get ready to start this transformative journey towards becoming healthy at home!

Chapter 1: Setting Your Goals

Alright, let's dive into the first step of your fitness journey: setting your goals. You might be wondering why this is so important, and trust me, it's a game-changer. Without clear goals, staying motivated and tracking your progress can feel like trying to find your way without a map. So, let's chat about why setting goals matters, the different types of goals you can set, and how to make sure your goals are effective.

Why Goal Setting Matters

Imagine starting a road trip without a destination. You'd probably end up driving around aimlessly, wasting time and gas. The same goes for fitness. Goals give you direction and purpose. They act as your roadmap, guiding you through the ups and downs of your fitness journey. When you know exactly what you're aiming for, it's much easier to stay focused and motivated, even when things get tough. Plus, having goals allows you to measure your progress and tweak your plan as needed.

Types of Goals

Now, let's talk about the two main types of fitness goals: outcome-based and process-based.

- **Outcome-based goals** are all about the end results you want. Think of these as your big-picture goals. Examples include losing a specific amount of weight, running a marathon, or fitting into a particular dress size. These goals are great for motivation because they give you something concrete to strive for.

- **Process-based goals**, on the other hand, focus on the daily or weekly actions you need to take to reach those big-picture goals. These might include working out a certain number of days per week, eating a balanced diet, or ensuring you get enough sleep. Process-based goals are crucial because they help you build the habits and behaviors necessary for long-term success.

S.M.A.R.T. Goals

To make your goals as effective as possible, you should use the S.M.A.R.T. framework. This stands for Specific, Measurable, Attainable, Relevant, and Time-based. Let's break it down:

- **Specific**: Your goals should be clear and detailed. Instead of saying, "I want to be fit," think about what being fit means to you. Maybe it's "I want to run a 5K without stopping."
- **Measurable**: Make sure you can track your progress. If your goal is to gain strength, you might aim to lift a certain weight within a specific timeframe.

- **Attainable**: Set realistic goals. It's great to aim high, but setting goals that are too far out of reach can lead to frustration. Make sure your goals challenge you but are still achievable.
- **Relevant**: Your goals should align with your values and priorities. They need to be important to you and positively impact your overall well-being.
- **Time-based**: Set a deadline. This adds a sense of urgency and helps keep you accountable. For example, instead of saying, "I want to lose weight," say, "I want to lose 10 pounds in three months."

Setting Your Goals

Now that you get the importance of goal setting and how to make your goals S.M.A.R.T., it's time to set your own fitness goals. Think about what you want to achieve. Is it weight loss, muscle gain, improved endurance, or increased flexibility? Write down your goals and ensure they align with your values and priorities. Make them specific, measurable, attainable, relevant, and time-based. Breaking them down into smaller milestones can make them more manageable and help you track your progress.

Conclusion

Setting goals is the foundation of a successful fitness journey. It gives you purpose, direction, and motivation. By making your goals S.M.A.R.T., you significantly increase your chances of success. Take the time to define your goals clearly, and use them as a guide to create a personalized and effective fitness plan.

Chapter 2: Creating Your Ideal Home Gym

Ready to set up your ideal home gym? This is such an exciting step in your fitness journey. Having a dedicated space where you can exercise and focus on your health can really make a difference in achieving your goals. Let's walk through how to design and set up the perfect home gym together.

Benefits of a Home Gym

First off, let's talk about why having a home gym is such a great idea. The benefits are pretty impressive. For starters, you eliminate the need to commute to a fitness center, which saves you both time and money. Plus, you have the convenience of exercising whenever you want, without worrying about gym hours or crowded spaces. Another huge advantage is that you can customize your gym to fit your specific fitness preferences and goals. And let's not forget the comfort and familiarity of working out at home, which can really boost your motivation and help you stay consistent.

Assessing Your Space

Before we dive into picking out equipment and figuring out the layout, it's essential to take a good look at the space you have available. Whether you've got a whole room to dedicate or just a corner of a room, understanding your space limitations will help you optimize its use. Start by taking measurements of the area. Consider the type of flooring you have—hardwood, carpet, or something else. Think about other factors that might impact your workouts, like low ceilings or limited ventilation. Knowing these details will help you plan a functional and comfortable gym setup.

Equipment Selection

Choosing the right equipment is a key part of creating an effective home gym. It's important to think about your fitness goals and the types of exercises you enjoy. Here are some essential equipment options to consider:

- **Cardio Machines**: Treadmills, stationary bikes, or ellipticals are great for getting your heart rate up.
- **Strength Training Equipment**: Dumbbells, resistance bands, kettlebells, or a weight bench will help you build muscle.
- **Functional Training Tools**: Stability balls, medicine balls, or TRX systems can add variety to your workouts.
- **Additional Accessories**: Yoga mats, foam rollers, jump ropes, or pull-up bars are versatile tools that enhance your routine.

Make sure the equipment you choose matches your current fitness level and aligns with your long-term goals. Also, think about how you'll store everything. Maybe you can use shelves, racks, or storage bins to keep your space organized.

Ergonomics and Safety

When you're setting up your home gym, ergonomics and safety should be top priorities. Arrange your equipment in a way that allows for smooth movement and minimizes the risk of injury. Ensure there's enough space to perform exercises comfortably and without restrictions. Mirrors on the walls can be a great addition because they let you check your form and technique. Also, investing in quality exercise mats can protect your joints and provide stability during your workouts.

Creating a Motivating Environment

Your home gym should be a place where you feel motivated and excited to work out. Consider painting the walls with energizing colors or hanging motivational quotes and posters. Good lighting is crucial, so make sure your gym is well-lit and vibrant. Music can be a powerful motivator, so set up a sound system or have a playlist ready to keep you pumped up during your workouts. The more inviting and personalized your gym space feels, the more likely you are to enjoy exercising and stick with it.

Conclusion

Creating your ideal home gym is a fun and rewarding process. By assessing your space, selecting the right equipment, prioritizing safety, and crafting a motivating environment, you can design a gym that fits your fitness goals and preferences perfectly. With your customized gym at your disposal, you'll be well on your way to achieving fitness success right from the comfort of your own home.

Chapter 3: Designing Effective Workouts

Alright, so now that you've got your home gym all set up, it's time to dive into designing workouts that will help you crush your fitness goals. This might seem a bit overwhelming, especially if you're new to fitness or unsure where to start. But don't worry, we're here to guide you through the process and give you the tools you need to create workouts that are both challenging and enjoyable.

Understanding Your Fitness Goals

First things first: let's talk about your fitness goals. Knowing what you want to achieve will shape how you design your workouts. Are you aiming to lose weight, build muscle, improve cardiovascular endurance, or increase flexibility? Each goal requires a slightly different approach, so identifying your primary objective is crucial.

The Components of a Well-Rounded Workout

A balanced workout includes several key components: cardiovascular exercise, strength training, flexibility work, and rest and recovery. Let's break these down a bit:

1. **Cardiovascular Exercise**

- Cardio is essential for improving heart health, burning calories, and boosting overall endurance. Think activities like jogging, cycling, swimming, jumping rope, or using cardio machines like treadmills and ellipticals. Find something you enjoy, as this will make it easier to stick with it.

2. **Strength Training**
   - Strength training helps build lean muscle mass, increase strength, and improve body composition. This involves using resistance, such as weights or resistance bands, to target specific muscle groups. Incorporate exercises like squats, lunges, push-ups, and dumbbell curls. Start with lighter weights and gradually increase as you get stronger.

3. **Flexibility Work**
   - Flexibility exercises are often overlooked but are crucial for overall fitness. They help improve your range of motion, prevent injuries, and reduce muscle soreness. Try to include dynamic stretches, static stretches, or yoga poses in your routine.

4. **Rest and Recovery**

o Rest and recovery are vital parts of any workout program. Your body needs time to repair and rebuild muscle tissue after intense exercise. Be sure to schedule rest days to allow for proper recovery. This will help you avoid burnout and keep your fitness journey sustainable.

Structuring Your Workouts

A well-structured workout has three main phases: warm-up, main workout, and cool-down. Let's take a closer look at each phase:

1. **Warm-up**
   o The warm-up is crucial for preparing your body for the main workout. It should include light cardiovascular exercises, like brisk walking or jogging, and dynamic stretching to loosen up your muscles. This helps prevent injuries and gets your body ready for more intense activity.
2. **Main Workout**
   o This is the core of your workout, where you focus on exercises that align with your fitness goals. Make sure to mix in cardio, strength training, and flexibility work. You might create a circuit-style workout, alternating between different

exercises, or follow a specific program tailored to your goals.

3. **Cool-down**
   - The cool-down phase helps your body gradually return to its resting state. Include gentle stretches to improve flexibility and reduce post-workout muscle soreness. Cooling down properly also helps prevent dizziness, lightheadedness, and injuries.

Progression and Variation

To keep making progress and avoid hitting plateaus, it's important to incorporate progression and variation into your workouts.

- **Progression** means gradually increasing the intensity, duration, or complexity of your workouts. This could be by adding more weight, increasing the number of repetitions or sets, or reducing rest time between exercises.
- **Variation** involves changing up your workouts regularly to keep your body challenged and prevent boredom. Try different exercises, use various equipment, switch up your workout formats, or even take different fitness classes.

Listen to Your Body

Lastly, always listen to your body. If you feel pain or discomfort during a workout, it's important to modify or stop the exercise. Muscle soreness is normal, but sharp or persistent pain should not be ignored. Prioritize rest and recovery to allow your body to heal and prevent overtraining.

Designing effective workouts is both a science and an art. It might take some trial and error to find what works best for you, but with the knowledge and guidelines provided in this chapter, you're well-equipped to create workouts that align with your fitness goals and keep you motivated on your home fitness journey.

Chapter 4: Mastering Exercise Form and Technique

Alright, let's talk about something really crucial for your fitness journey: mastering exercise form and technique. Whether you're just starting out or you've been working out for years, performing exercises correctly is key to getting the best results and avoiding injuries. Let's dive into why this matters and how you can ensure you're doing it right.

The Importance of Proper Form

You might wonder why proper form is such a big deal. Well, when you do exercises with the correct form, you engage the right muscles more effectively. This not only helps you achieve better muscle development and overall strength, but it also minimizes the stress on your joints and reduces the risk of injury. Think of it this way: if you're lifting weights with poor form, you might be putting unnecessary strain on your back or knees, which can lead to problems down the line.

Focusing on Core Stability

One of the foundations of good exercise form is core stability. Your core isn't just your abs—it includes muscles in your abdomen, back, hips, and pelvis. A strong core provides a stable base for movement and helps transfer force between your upper and lower body. By focusing on strengthening your core, you'll improve your overall physical performance and lower your risk of injuries.

Guidelines for Correct Exercise Form

To help you nail down proper form and technique, here are some guidelines to follow:

1. **Start with Proper Alignment**
    - Before you even begin an exercise, make sure your body is properly aligned. Stand tall with your shoulders down and back, chest lifted, and spine in a neutral position. This sets a solid foundation for any movement.
2. **Engage the Targeted Muscles**
    - Focus on engaging the muscles you intend to work during each exercise. This means consciously activating the targeted muscle group, ensuring you're using the right muscles for the right movements.
3. **Control Your Movements**
    - Slow and controlled movements are your best friend. Avoid jerking or using momentum to complete the exercise. The more controlled your movements, the more effective

they'll be in targeting the desired
muscle groups.

4. **Use the Full Range of Motion**
    - Perform each exercise through its
      full range of motion. Don't cut
      corners or shorten the movement.
      This allows for maximum muscle
      activation and helps develop
      flexibility.

5. **Breathe Properly**
    - Remember to breathe! Inhale during
      the easier part of the movement and
      exhale during the more challenging
      phase. Proper breathing helps
      stabilize your core and keeps you
      focused.

6. **Seek Professional Guidance**
    - If you're unsure about your form or
      technique, consider consulting a
      certified personal trainer or fitness
      professional. They can provide
      expert guidance and help correct
      any form errors, ensuring you're
      performing exercises safely and
      effectively.

Why This All Matters

Mastering exercise form and technique isn't just
about looking good while you work out. It's about
making sure you're getting the most out of your
efforts and keeping your body safe. When you take

the time to learn and practice proper form, you're setting yourself up for success in the long run. Your workouts will be more efficient, you'll see better results, and you'll avoid the pitfalls of improper technique, like injuries that could set you back.

So, let's put this into practice. Next time you're in your home gym, take a few extra minutes to focus on your form. Watch yourself in a mirror, record a video for self-review, or even better, get some feedback from a professional. Over time, these small adjustments will become second nature, and you'll be well on your way to safer, more effective workouts. Keep at it, and you'll reap the rewards of all your hard work.

Chapter 5: Optimizing Nutrition for Fitness

Alright, let's dive into the delicious world of nutrition and see how it can turbocharge your fitness journey. Eating right isn't just about fueling your body for workouts—it's about supporting your overall health, aiding in recovery, and helping you build that lean muscle you've been working hard for. So, let's chat about how you can optimize your nutrition to make the most out of your fitness efforts.

The Role of Nutrition in Fitness

Think of nutrition as the backbone of your fitness routine. Without the right nutrients, your body won't perform at its best. Good nutrition helps you power through workouts, recover faster, build muscle, and maintain overall well-being. By giving your body the fuel it needs, you can boost your performance, enhance your stamina, and reach your fitness goals more efficiently.

Understanding Macronutrients and Micronutrients

To get the most out of your diet, you need to understand macronutrients (carbohydrates, proteins, and fats) and micronutrients (vitamins and minerals).

1. Carbohydrates Carbs are your body's main source of energy. They power your workouts and help replenish glycogen stores in your muscles. But not all carbs are created equal. Opt for complex carbohydrates like whole grains, fruits, and vegetables. These provide sustained energy and essential nutrients that keep you going strong.

2. Proteins Proteins are the building blocks of your muscles. They're crucial for muscle repair and growth. Make sure to include lean protein sources in your diet, such as chicken, fish, tofu, beans, and legumes. These foods will help you build and maintain muscle mass, which is key for a strong and fit body.

3. Fats Healthy fats are essential for hormone production, brain function, and energy. Don't shy away from fats—instead, choose the right kinds. Incorporate sources of omega-3 fatty acids like fatty fish, avocados, nuts, and seeds. These healthy fats support various bodily functions and keep you energized.

4. Vitamins and Minerals Vitamins and minerals might not get as much attention, but they're vital for overall health. They support everything from immune function to bone health. Make sure your diet includes a variety of fruits, vegetables, whole grains, and lean proteins to meet your daily requirements.

Hydration

Don't forget about hydration! Proper hydration is crucial for digestion, nutrient absorption, muscle function, and temperature regulation. Drink plenty of water throughout the day, especially before, during, and after your workouts. Staying hydrated ensures your body operates at peak efficiency.

Eating for Energy and Recovery

Strategic eating around your workouts can make a big difference. Before you hit the gym, have a balanced meal that includes carbs for energy and protein to support muscle repair. After your workout, focus on replenishing glycogen stores and aiding recovery with protein and carbs. This helps your body bounce back and get ready for the next session.

Meal Planning and Portion Control

Meal planning and portion control are your allies in sticking to your nutrition goals. Plan your meals ahead of time to ensure they're balanced and nutrient-rich. Using portion control techniques can help you manage your calorie intake and maintain a healthy weight. It's all about finding a routine that works for you and sticking to it.

Supplements

While getting nutrients from whole foods is ideal, sometimes supplements can help fill in the gaps. If you think you might need supplements, consult with a healthcare professional or a registered dietitian. They can provide guidance based on your specific fitness goals and nutritional needs.

Conclusion

Optimizing your nutrition is a game-changer for your fitness journey. By focusing on the right balance of macronutrients and micronutrients, staying hydrated, and planning your meals wisely, you can enhance your performance and support your overall health. Don't forget to listen to your body and seek professional advice when needed.

Chapter 6: Incorporating Functional Fitness

Alright, let's talk about functional fitness. It's a game-changer when it comes to making your workouts not just effective but also relevant to everyday life. Imagine being able to carry groceries, pick up your kids, or even reach that top shelf without straining yourself. That's the magic of functional fitness—exercises that mimic real-life movements to boost your strength, balance, flexibility, and coordination. Let's dive in and see how you can incorporate this into your home workout routine.

Understanding Functional Fitness

Functional fitness focuses on exercises that improve your ability to perform everyday activities with ease. These movements are practical and applicable to daily life. Think about the motions you go through every day: lifting, squatting, pulling, pushing, and bending. By integrating these types of movements into your workouts, you're training your body to handle daily tasks more efficiently and safely.

The Benefits of Functional Fitness

Incorporating functional fitness into your routine comes with a slew of benefits. Here's why you should consider it:

1. Improved Functional Strength
Functional exercises work multiple muscle groups simultaneously, helping you develop strength that translates to real-life movements. This means you're not just getting stronger but also more capable in everyday activities.

2. Enhanced Balance and Stability
Many functional exercises engage your core and require you to stabilize your body, which boosts your balance and stability. This is especially important as you age, to prevent falls and maintain mobility.

3. Increased Flexibility and Mobility
Functional fitness often includes exercises that improve your range of motion, helping to prevent injuries and reduce joint pain. This makes daily activities, like bending and reaching, much easier.

4. Better Coordination and Agility
Exercises that challenge your coordination and agility can improve your ability to perform complex movements and react quickly, making you more adept at handling unexpected situations.

5. Increased Calorie Burn
Because functional exercises engage multiple muscles and movements, they tend to burn more

calories than isolated exercises. This can be a great advantage if weight loss is one of your goals.

6. Time-Efficient Workouts

Functional exercises target several areas of fitness at once, allowing you to maximize your workout time. You can achieve a lot more in a shorter period, which is perfect for busy schedules.

Incorporating Functional Fitness into Your Home Workout

Ready to start? Here's how you can integrate functional fitness into your home workouts:

1. Choose Functional Exercises

Look for exercises that mimic everyday movements and use multiple muscle groups. Some great examples include squats, lunges, push-ups, planks, and kettlebell swings. These exercises not only build strength but also enhance your movement patterns.

2. Use Unstable Surfaces

Incorporating tools like balance boards or Bosu balls can add an extra challenge to your exercises, improving your balance and stability. This helps you develop better control over your body in various conditions.

3. Focus on Functional Strength

Select exercises that strengthen the muscles you

use most frequently in daily activities. For instance, if you often carry heavy objects, focus on strengthening your legs, core, and upper body with exercises like deadlifts, squats, and shoulder presses.

4. Incorporate Functional Training Tools

Adding resistance bands, medicine balls, or suspension trainers to your home gym can diversify your workouts and provide additional resistance. These tools can simulate real-life resistance and enhance your overall strength.

5. Balance Cardio and Strength

While functional exercises can offer cardiovascular benefits, it's important to balance them with dedicated cardio exercises such as jogging, cycling, or jumping rope. This ensures a well-rounded fitness routine.

6. Progress Gradually

Start with exercises that match your current fitness level and gradually increase the intensity, duration, and complexity. This approach helps prevent injuries and ensures steady progress. Listen to your body and give it time to adapt.

Sample Functional Workout

To get you started, here's a sample functional workout that you can try at home:

Warm-up

- **Light Cardio:** 5-10 minutes of jogging in place or jumping jacks to get your heart rate up and muscles warmed.

Main Workout

- **Goblet Squats:** 3 sets of 12 reps
- **Push-ups:** 3 sets of 10 reps
- **Standing Rows with Resistance Band:** 3 sets of 12 reps
- **Plank:** Hold for 30 seconds, rest for 15 seconds, repeat 3 times
- **Step-ups with Dumbbells:** 3 sets of 10 reps per leg

Cool-down

- **Stretching:** 5-10 minutes of stretching to relax and lengthen your muscles. Focus on areas that were worked the most during your session.

Remember, you can adjust this workout based on your fitness level. If you're just starting out, reduce the number of sets or reps, and gradually increase them as you get stronger. And if you're ever unsure about your form or how to progress, don't hesitate to consult a fitness professional.

Conclusion

Incorporating functional fitness into your home workouts is a fantastic way to enhance your physical function and overall well-being. By focusing on exercises that mimic everyday movements and utilizing functional training tools, you'll build strength, balance, flexibility, and coordination. Just remember to progress gradually and consult with a professional if needed.

Chapter 7: Staying Motivated and Consistent

Staying motivated and consistent on your fitness journey can be a challenge, but it's essential for achieving your goals and maintaining a healthy lifestyle. Let's chat about some strategies that can help you stay on track and keep pushing forward, even when things get tough.

1. Set Clear Goals

First and foremost, you need to set clear and specific goals. Think about what you want to achieve: is it losing weight, building muscle, or improving your overall fitness level? Make sure your goals are measurable and attainable. For example, instead of just saying "I want to lose weight," aim for "I want to lose 10 pounds in three months." Break down these long-term goals into smaller, manageable milestones you can work towards daily or weekly. This way, you'll get a sense of accomplishment regularly, which will keep you motivated.

2. Find Your Why

Understanding your "why" is crucial. Ask yourself why you're pursuing these fitness goals. Is it to improve your health, boost your confidence, or set an example for your kids? Whatever your reasons, keep them in mind. When your motivation starts to fade, remind yourself of these reasons. Your "why" can be a powerful motivator on tough days.

3. Create a Supportive Environment

Having a supportive environment can make all the difference. Share your goals with friends and family who can cheer you on. Join online fitness communities or local support groups. Finding a workout buddy can also be incredibly helpful. This way, you have someone to hold you accountable and share your journey with. Support from others can provide the encouragement you need when you're feeling down.

4. Mix Up Your Routine

Doing the same workout routine every day can get boring quickly. Keep things fresh and exciting by mixing up your exercises. Try new activities like yoga, pilates, cycling, or even hiking. Variety not only keeps you engaged but also challenges different muscle groups, preventing plateaus and keeping your workouts effective.

5. Set Realistic Expectations

It's essential to set realistic expectations for yourself. Understand that progress takes time and won't happen overnight. Be patient and focus on the small wins along the way. Celebrate these little victories, whether it's running an extra mile or lifting heavier weights. Each small step forward is a step closer to your ultimate goal.

6. Track Your Progress

Keeping track of your progress can be incredibly motivating. Use a workout journal or a fitness app to record your workouts, measurements, and achievements. Seeing your progress in black and white can be a great reminder of how far you've come, motivating you to keep pushing forward.

7. Reward Yourself

Rewards can be a great way to boost motivation. Set up a reward system for reaching milestones or achieving specific goals. Treat yourself to something special, like a massage, a new workout outfit, or a night out with friends. These rewards can make your fitness journey more enjoyable and give you something to look forward to.

8. Be Flexible and Adapt

Life happens, and sometimes your original workout plan might not be feasible. Be flexible and ready to adapt. If time is tight, opt for shorter, more intense workouts. If you're traveling, find ways to exercise on the go. The key is to stay committed, even if it means adjusting your routine to fit your current situation.

9. Practice Self-Care

Taking care of your physical and mental well-being is crucial. Make time for rest and recovery, get quality sleep, and eat nutritious foods. Incorporate stress-reducing activities like meditation, yoga, or even just a relaxing bath. When you feel good physically and mentally, you'll be more motivated to stick with your fitness routine.

10. Celebrate Your Success

Finally, don't forget to celebrate your successes, both big and small. Acknowledge your achievements and reward yourself. Share your progress with your support system and reflect on how far you've come. Celebrating your success not only boosts your motivation but also reinforces your commitment to a healthy lifestyle.

By implementing these strategies, you can stay motivated and consistent on your fitness journey. Remember, motivation may ebb and flow, but by staying focused, adapting to challenges, and maintaining a positive mindset, you can overcome any obstacles. Stay dedicated, believe in yourself, and enjoy the journey to becoming a healthier and stronger version of yourself.

Chapter 8: Prioritizing Recovery and Self-Care

Hey there, fellow fitness enthusiast! Welcome to a crucial chapter in your fitness journey: prioritizing recovery and self-care. You know, while crushing those workouts in your home gym is fantastic, it's equally essential to give your body and mind the TLC they deserve. So, let's dive into some strategies and techniques that'll help you recover like a champ and nurture yourself along the way.

The Importance of Recovery

Alright, let's get real about recovery. It's not just about lounging on the couch (although that's pretty nice too!). Recovery is crucial for your body to recharge its batteries, repair those hard-working muscles, and optimize your performance. Skipping out on recovery can lead to overtraining, muscle imbalances, and even mental burnout. Here's why it's a big deal:

1. **Reduced Risk of Injuries:** Taking time to rest and recover gives your muscles and joints the chance to repair and strengthen, lowering the risk of pesky injuries.
2. **Improved Muscle Growth and Strength:** When you rest, your muscles rebuild and grow stronger, leading to better performance and gains.

3. **Enhanced Mental Well-Being:** Recovery time allows you to recharge mentally, reducing stress levels and boosting your mood.
4. **Better Sleep Quality:** Prioritizing recovery can also improve the quality of your sleep, which is vital for muscle repair and overall health.

Now that we've got the lowdown on why recovery matters, let's explore some killer strategies to weave into your routine.

Rest and Active Recovery

Rest days are like the VIP lounge for your muscles. They're essential for proper recovery and growth. But rest doesn't always mean doing nothing. You can opt for active recovery activities like gentle stretching, yoga, or low-intensity exercises such as walking or swimming. These keep the blood flowing and help ease muscle soreness.

Nutrition for Recovery

You can't out-train a bad diet, right? Proper nutrition is key for recovery. Load up on protein to support muscle repair and growth. Think lean meats, fish, eggs, tofu, and legumes. Don't forget about carbs to replenish those glycogen stores and provide energy. Whole grains, fruits, and veggies are your best pals here. And, of course, stay hydrated like it's your job.

Quality Sleep

Ah, the magic of sleep! Aim for seven to nine hours of quality shut-eye each night. Establish a bedtime routine, create a cozy sleep environment, and ditch those screens before bed. Your body and mind will thank you for it.

Self-Care Practices

It's not all about physical recovery; mental rejuvenation is just as vital. Treat yourself to some self-care activities like stretching, meditation, or even a hot bath. Journaling, spending time in nature, or getting a massage are also excellent options. Find what speaks to your soul and make it a regular part of your routine.

Creating a Balanced Routine

Finding the sweet spot between challenging workouts and ample recovery time is key. Listen to your body, adjust your workouts as needed, and don't skimp on rest days. Remember, it's better to take it slow and steady than to risk burnout or injury.

Conclusion

Alright, friend, here's the bottom line: prioritizing recovery and self-care isn't just a luxury—it's a necessity for a kickass fitness routine. By giving your body and mind the love they deserve, you'll optimize your results and ensure long-term well-being. So, go ahead, incorporate rest, good nutrition, quality sleep, and self-care practices into your life. Your body will thank you, and your fitness journey will be all the better for it.

Chapter 9: Tracking Progress and Celebrating Success

Hey there, fitness warrior! Strap in because we're diving into a crucial chapter of your fitness journey: tracking your progress and celebrating those hard-earned wins. Trust me, this is the fun part!

Why Track Your Progress?

Alright, let's talk about why tracking progress is a game-changer. Firstly, it's like having your own personal cheerleader shouting, "You got this!" Seeing those little victories—whether it's pumping out extra reps or shaving seconds off your run—can light a fire under you like nothing else. Plus, it gives you concrete evidence that your sweat sessions are paying off.

Secondly, tracking your progress helps you spot any roadblocks ahead. If you're not seeing the gains you expected, it's your cue to adjust your game plan. Maybe you need to switch up your workouts or tweak your nutrition. Tracking keeps you one step ahead of plateaus and setbacks.

Lastly, it keeps you grounded. By knowing where you're at, you can set realistic goals that actually light you up. No more aiming for the stars and crashing back to earth—it's all about steady, achievable progress.

Methods of Tracking Progress

So, how do you track your fitness journey like a pro? Here are a few methods to consider:

1. **Fitness Journals:** Think of it as your workout diary. Jot down your exercises, sets, reps, and how you felt during your sweat sesh. It's like having a roadmap of your fitness journey right at your fingertips.
2. **Technology and Apps:** Hello, digital age! There are tons of fitness apps and devices out there that make tracking a breeze. Whether it's steps taken, calories burned, or heart rate, these apps do the heavy lifting for you.
3. **Body Measurements:** Who needs a scale when you've got a tape measure? Track changes in your waist, hips, and other key areas to get the full picture of your progress. Remember, it's not just about the number on the scale!

Celebrating Success

Now, let's talk about the fun part: celebrating those victories, big and small. Here's how to make every win count:

1. **Reward Yourself:** Hit a milestone? Treat yourself! Whether it's a spa day, a new pair

of kicks, or a guilt-free cheat meal, rewards keep that motivation train chugging along.

2. **Share Your Success:** Don't keep those gains to yourself! Share your achievements with your squad—whether it's on social media or in your group chat. Their high-fives and fist bumps will keep you riding that wave of success.

3. **Set New Goals:** You did it once, now do it again! Set new goals that challenge and excite you. Whether it's lifting heavier, running faster, or mastering a new move, keep that momentum going.

4. **Reflect and Appreciate:** Take a moment to bask in your glory. Look back at how far you've come, from those shaky first reps to crushing your PRs. You've put in the work, so own it!

Conclusion

There you have it, fitness rockstar: tracking your progress and celebrating your success is the secret sauce to a killer fitness journey. By keeping tabs on your gains and giving yourself a pat on the back, you'll stay motivated, smash your goals, and become the superhero version of yourself you've always dreamed of. So, keep tracking, keep celebrating, and keep kicking butt! You've got this.

Chapter 10: Living Your Best Life: Embracing Holistic Health

Hey there, wellness warrior! Welcome to the final chapter of your journey to fitness greatness. Today, we're diving deep into the world of holistic health and exploring why it's essential to embrace a lifestyle that goes beyond just hitting the gym.

What's a Healthy Lifestyle Anyway?

Alright, let's break it down. A healthy lifestyle isn't just about sweating it out on the treadmill—it's a whole vibe. We're talking about nailing your nutrition, catching those Z's, managing stress like a boss, and showing yourself some serious self-love. It's the whole package, baby!

Let's Talk Nutrition

We've already hammered home the importance of good grub for your gains, but it's worth repeating. Eating right isn't just about choking down kale salads—it's about nourishing your body with the good stuff. Load up on fruits, veggies, lean proteins, and healthy fats, and skip the crash diets in favor of sustainable eating habits. And hey, if you're feeling lost in the sea of nutrition info out there, don't be afraid to call in the big guns—a registered dietitian can help steer you in the right direction.

Sleep, Sweet Sleep

Ah, the sweet sound of snoozing. Sleep isn't just for catching Z's—it's a crucial part of staying on top of your game. Clocking in those seven to nine hours isn't just a suggestion—it's a non-negotiable. So, dim those lights, cozy up in bed, and get ready to recharge like a boss.

Stress Less, Live More

In a world that never seems to slow down, stress is the silent killer of good vibes. But fear not, because you've got the tools to fight back. Whether it's deep breathing, downward dogging, or diving into your favorite hobby, finding ways to chill out is key to staying sane in this crazy world.

Self-Care, Because You're Worth It

Repeat after me: self-love is not selfish. Taking care of numero uno isn't just okay—it's essential. So, pencil in that bubble bath, dust off your journal, or treat yourself to a little TLC. Your mind, body, and soul will thank you for it.

Building Healthy Connections

They say you're the average of the five people you spend the most time with, so choose wisely! Surrounding yourself with positive peeps who lift you up is crucial for staying on track with your goals. Whether it's hitting the gym with your workout buddy or sharing a laugh with your bestie, lean on your squad for support and good vibes.

Balance, Baby

Listen up, my friend: life's too short to be stuck in extremes. Finding that sweet spot between kale smoothies and cheat days is where the magic happens. So, go ahead—indulge in that chocolate cake, take a rest day guilt-free, and remember that balance is the name of the game.

Celebrate the Wins, Big and Small

Last but not least, it's time to celebrate! Every PR smashed, every healthy meal devoured, every stress-busting yoga sesh—it all deserves a round of applause. Treat yourself to something special, shout your achievements from the rooftops, and take a moment to bask in the glory of how far you've come.

Conclusion: Here's to You, Health Hero!

And there you have it, my friend: the ultimate guide to living your best life. By embracing holistic health, you're not just crushing your fitness goals—you're taking charge of your entire existence. So keep fueling your body with the good stuff, catching those Z's, and showing yourself some serious love. You're a wellness warrior, and the world is your playground. Cheers to you and your journey to greatness!

www.ingramcontent.com/pod-product-compliance
Lightning Source LLC
Chambersburg PA
CBHW051855250726
48659CB00006B/2230